Table of Contents

Exploring the Causes and Treatment of Upper Back Pain

Exploring the Relationship Between Upper Back Pain and Cancer

1. Introduction to Upper Back Pain and Cancer

Only a subset of patients at the onset of pain is due to tumor injury and a signal referred to physicians assists in locating patients who are likely to have a cancer that needs to be diagnosed. Some characteristics will suggest that an X-ray should be performed. From here, the healing process is noted. As yet, a back pain cancer research group has not yet unified into one program. Furthermore, little or no scientific relationship between back pain and cancer has been established and presented in the best sound scientific literature. Most evidence is based on expert opinion, investigation, and narrative reviews. In a way, it highlights the significance of conducting cancer research.

One of the incredible features of the human body is the pain that warns of possible injuries or illness. Due to wear and tear in our bodies, severe pain can happen in different areas. An example of pain is upper back pain. Upper back pain refers to pain that occurs between the neck and bottom of the rib cage. The pain can vary from a dull ache to sharp pain. Patients with back pain have always been challenging, and all other diseases and conditions can mimic back pain. Cancer is frequently listed alongside common causes. Different types of cancer are often listed as possible causes. The pathophysiology of pain in cancer is known to range widely and depends on the type of cancer. Apart from that, some common causes of upper back pain are infections, poor posture, overuse, osteoarthritis, and thoracic spine diseases, just to mention a few symptoms. In general, the fact that a variety of conditions can lead to upper back pain has long been acknowledged.

2. Anatomy and Causes of Upper Back Pain

The causes of upper back pain can be just as expansive as its anatomy. Most often, upper back pain is of mechanical origin, commonly standing alone as an isolated, incidental complaint resulting from some sudden increase in demand or some awkward, bulging, or repetitive force. In such instances, cartilage tears (anular tears), herniations of the spinal discs, and change- or overuse-related disruption or damage to the muscular core often underpin the patient's pain. Articular degeneration of the facet joints can lead to joint pain, usually referred to as facet arthropathy, where pain is typically more prevalent on one side than the other. Other times, pain lower in the back can move up, in a sense reverberating off some structural brick within the lower spine. Oftentimes, the building blocks of the spine react in unnatural ways, causing pain and disability for patients throughout the spine, with the upper back being no exception.

The anatomy of upper back pain is vast. The upper back, also known as the thoracic spine, consists of 12 vertebrae or the bony building blocks of the spine, each numbered according to its position and corresponding nerve root. In between the spinous processes of these vertebrae, which are the bony tubes a doctor can actually feel when palpating a spine, exists a network of ligaments, tendons, and individual muscles, including the oft-maligned rhomboids, serratus muscles, latissimus dorsi, and trapezius, to name a few. The ribs cover the front and some of the back of the thoracic spine, forming the chest cavity and protecting vital organs, like the heart and lungs. There are three major joints between the ribs and the vertebrae, which make up the costovertebral articulation, providing the majority of mobility for the upper thoracic spine. Further, the upper back curves slightly into kyphosis, a reverse curvature to the direction of lordosis, the curve of the lower back.

3. Types of Cancer Associated with Upper Back Pain

Upper back pain is one of the symptoms that could be a sign of lung cancer. Back pain, in general, has many potential causes: there are several diseases and conditions associated with backache. Tumors that spread (metastasize) to the spine and compress the bones and nerves surrounding the vertebrae can cause back pain in lung cancer. People with lung cancer and back pain generally have severe pain. Spinal cord compression may occur; this condition presents as tingling, numbness, or weakness in one or both feet. Pancreatic cancer is another source of upper back pain. Pancreatic cancer can cause pain in the mid-to-upper abdomen and back. It has typically spread by the time it is diagnosed - often to the liver. Breast cancer that results in the spread of cancer cells to the bone causes upper back pain. Metastatic lesions in other cancers can also result in back pain, sometimes described as severe, while the muscles are usually affected. If you have severe pain, compression effects may be occurring, and tumors that usually compress vertebrae also affect bone tissue. Pain generally intensifies at night.

Upper back pain is directly related to lung cancer. This is because lung tumors directly compress the vertebrae and tissues in their vicinity, which can cause severe backache. While pain is a common symptom of cancer, fatigue and unintended weight loss are other typical symptoms of most cancers. Investigations such as X-rays, MRI, or a CT scan are also conducted because lungs are located in the chest region. Upper thoracic cancer can also result in upper back pain. Unlike bone-related pain, muscle-related pain is usually not severe. Breast cancer can spread to bone, and this can cause upper back pain. A tell-tale sign is an occurrence of pain that is worse at night or that has been documented to occur at night. On the other hand, pain in the upper back region is another typical sign of pancreatic cancer. Respiratory symptoms include coughing up blood, a persistent cough, and shortness of breath. Pain is another common symptom of lung cancer and can result from metastases to most chest locations.

3.1. Lung Cancer

Damage to the cells initiates scar tissue formation in the area where the tumor is growing and can eventually press against the structures mentioned. The surrounding muscles and tissues begin to signal that a discomfort or pain which it "feels/interprets" as being local to the area where it comes into contact. This is the body's early strategy to alert the person to a potential problem. Diagnosis of cancer is most commonly confirmed by the presentation of an abnormal CT scan (the standard screening tool) and other imaging tools, like PET or MRI, used to evaluate more serious/denser tissues. Although lung cancer starts to spread in Stage 3B, it can cause pain only when there is significant disruption, dislodging, or "breaking off" from the main tumor. If the vertebra is significantly involved and radiation to stop this is not an option, then chemotherapy may be considered. If the vertebra is not involved and no spinal cord compression is present, surgical treatment of the lung cancer may be advised to ease the spreading of the tumor.

Lung cancer. Pain caused by cancer in any area of the body can be linked to a growing tumor pressing against nerves, organs, or the structure of the body. As described by Slater et al., lung cancer is one of the malignancies that propagates beyond the stroma in a matter of years, including the upper back area. The posterior aspect of the chest wall is an area that is somewhat sensitive to pain, with many visceral complaints presenting with some variation of referred shoulder pain along the upper back.

When a lung tumor reaches Stage 3B, it has spread to other parts of the chest and may affect other areas surrounding the lungs. This may include surrounding structures such as the esophagus, spine, pleura, ribs, chest wall, etc. It presents with at least one of the following signs or symptoms: it involves the main airways into the lungs, causing symptoms such as shortness of breath and cough; and lung cancer directly beneath the breastbones, and cancers that signal Horner's syndrome (tumor in the chest pressing on some nerves).

3.2. Breast Cancer

This paper provides a literature review on the association between upper back pain and breast cancer. The structure of this review reflects the findings of previous research on this theme. Typically, large databases, such as PubMed, Ovid, and Scopus, have been used to find such research. Tools employed included keywords (e.g., 'upper back pain', 'breast cancer', and 'spinal metastasis') and medical subject heading (MeSH) (e.g., 'Breast Neoplasm' and 'spinal metastasis'). Besides examining the relationship between upper back pain and breast cancer, this review addresses the specific factors contributing to upper back pain in individuals with breast cancer and proposes unique mechanisms and sources of back pain in this cohort. Also, an analysis of the typical diagnostic pathway and interventional treatments for upper back pain, with insights into particular diagnostic and treatment preferences, in women with breast cancer is included.

The breast cancer subsection is divided into two main parts. The first part is focused on non-invasive breast cancer, and the second part is focused on invasive breast cancer. Regarding the former, we suggest that troublesome back pain in these patients is typically due to the general muscular or skeletal aches and pains that can occur in men of this age, rather than a direct consequence of non-invasive machines or surgery. The one exception to this relates to those men treated with aromatase inhibitors, for whom osteoporosis is a long-term side effect that might need to be actively managed. In the second part of the section, we discuss the relationship between invasive breast cancer, biopsy and treatment-induced neuropathic pain syndromes, and more concerning bony metastases which can occur on a background of either intermittent or chronic back pain. Though unusual, the final subsection also considers rarer causes of breast cancer which may be more specific to men than women.

3.3. Pancreatic Cancer

In conclusion, pancreatic cancer is a common site of metastatic adenocarcinoma and passes through lymphatic spread and hematologic spread, mostly involving the liver. Due to direct extension, it can also involve structures of the GI system as well as surrounding vessels, leading to pain. Despite statistics supporting the presence of abdominal and epigastric pain in almost 50% of patients, 2/3 of those patients with alcohol etiology reported to have back pain. The back pain increasingly becomes the only symptom as the cancer progresses to late stages and is also the most common associated symptom definitive of pancreatic cancer. Upper back pain is due to the connection of the pancreas to the spine, resulting in the radiation of back pain. Research for interventional treatment, especially palliative care for pancreatic cancer, is limited, with nutrition supplementation, opioids, and opioids in combination with spinal ablation being the most effective. Pancreatic cancer therefore represents a unique battleground for the modern interventional pain physician, as most of the usual threats and dangers that the pancreas can signal are scientifically unimportant. However, the relationship may not be as strong as the association of a widened mediastinum with pancreatic cancer. In such instances, an ear for the uncommon can be life-saving.

Pancreatic cancer has been associated with upper back pain. Pancreatic cancer extends rapidly and may reach the nerves that connect at the spinal cord, thus causing back pain. Pain associated with pancreatic cancer also involves chemical substances released by the cancer that activate pain receptors. Failure to recognize the significance of back pain as a symptom of pancreatic cancer can lead to a lack of follow-up or misdiagnosis. Pain may arise before and during the progression of the disease and may persist after treatment. Several treatment options and interventional procedures are available for back pain, but the choice of procedure should be made in consultation with the patient's oncologist.

Pancreatic Neoplasm/Pancreatic Cancer

4. Mechanisms of Pain in Cancer Patients

Context/purpose: Pain is a subjective perception and a dominant fear staged by the patients. Intractable pain or incurable pain may be perceivable by the signals driven to peripheral nervous endings due to different pathological causes, as well as may occur only with psychosocial issues of the neurological transmission system.

Pain mechanisms and sensation mechanisms elucidated in detail cost billions of dollars still today, as long as it is quite difficult to address the mechanisms of the subjective complaints a patient is declaring. Cancer pain subjected to certain mechanisms is affected by the alterations on the injured or intact peripheral tissues, leading to variations in the functional state of the nervous system, changing the balance of the excitation and inhibition of spinal cord neurons and the synaptic and nonsynaptic processes, thereby modifying afferent signals transmitted to the central nervous system.

Pain mechanisms and sensation are complex in cancer patients, indicating that neuropathic, nociceptive, and psychological variables concurrently may have an effect on cancer pain, as well as the performance status of the patient. Cancer is the second or third most common cause of mortality for almost all countries worldwide. As long as methods of treatment have been developed through the recent years, cancer-related pain has been one of the first meaningful issues to address for treatment strategies in medical oncology centers. That being said, still today more than half of the cancer patients feel pain categorized as moderate to severe.

5. Diagnostic Approaches for Identifying Cancer-Related Back Pain

Apart from radiologic findings (alone or in combination), the determination of (actual) pain and/or neurology consistency with the anatomic/radiologic findings may be imperative as well, thereby supposedly increasing the "positive predictive value" of the latter. In summary, medical history-oriented/relevant questions and clinical examination as well as potentially blood markers may thus help to differentiate causes of back pain. Furthermore, in those where cancer is a potential risk, radiological tests (e.g., MRI, CT-scan; possibly whole-body imaging), if needed, should concentrate on spinal disease(s) to assist differential diagnosis for treatment and prognosis.

At a cost, MRI scans are very sensitive (i.e., they detect or recognize the vast majority of cancerous changes). As a result, MRI often "over-diagnoses" other conditions (i.e., it shows irregularities but doesn't show if they are really cancer-related or not) as well. Furthermore, MRI lacks the potential to identify (i.e., has false-negatives) or almost exclusive myeloma. As such, the trade-off between "sensitivity" and "specificity" for the (overall) detection of cancer relativity can be hazardous (i.e., "over-diagnosing" trivial radiologic lesions/irregularities while "missing" or "under-diagnosing" the actually relevant ones).

Diagnostic approaches to ascertain whether back pain is due to cancer rather than due to non-cancerous conditions may include: imaging methods (e.g., MRI of the relevant body part, positron emission topography), certain forms of blood tests (e.g., levels of specific markers, inflammation markers), and clinical assessments (e.g., physical examination, functional status, clinical questions). To help exclude (or possibly diagnose) cancer-related back pain - with possible involvement of cancer types other than myeloma - these tests can also be helpful.

6. Treatment Options for Cancer-Related Back Pain

Although opioids are frequently the front-line agents in the management of cancer pain and its associated back pain, other non-opioid pain medications – including acetaminophen, NSAIDs, antiepileptics, and TCAs – have been incorporated into clinical guidelines to provide maximum pain relief while minimizing dependency on opioid drugs. In addition to pharmacological treatments, non-pharmacological treatment options (exercise, acupuncture, heating pad) have been shown to be effective in managing back pain in the general population, and therefore would be a potential avenue to consider in the cancer treatment regimens. Furthermore, interventional procedures, including radiation therapy and local anesthetic agents, in the treatment of back pain have an increased role in the oncological setting, while surgical intervention can be useful in the management of spinal cord compression. Administration of antiresorptive agents as treatment or prevention of skeletal-related events – common in patients with back pain due to cancer – is common, particularly in patients with osseous metastasis. Radiation treatment is the preferred treatment for osseous metastasis followed by radioactive strontium. Bisphosphonates and PTH medication are used in patients with favorable performance status and solid tumor for the treatment of osseous metastasis management. Bone modifying agents are more suitable for use in patients with multiple myeloma for reducing the risk of skeletal-related events in the treatment of osseous metastasis. Reconstructive surgery is the same in patients with back pain due to osseous metastasis. Radiotherapy/Hospice treatment options should be treated in the following possible interventions. Rehabilitation, opioids, antidepressants, epidural steroid injections, procuring therapy, interventional injections, acupuncture, spine surgeries can be preferred treatment modalities for back pain management besides considering different treatment modalities, including musculoskeletal pain, and non-musculoskeletal back pain with cancer patients who are in an advanced stage of cancer.

One of the most important aspects in the management of cancer patients is to help in the relief of their symptoms. Back pain is one of the most common complaints encountered by healthcare professionals. There are many treatment options to help manage back pain. This involves using psychological pain management tools, medications, interventional/surgical procedures, and physiotherapy. The psychological part of pain relief is a very important part of the pain problems seen in this patient population. Treatment with medications usually involves prescribing more than one drug, and drug combinations are available or used to achieve the best outcome. Non-pharmacological treatment options can be used and include early physical therapy and rehabilitation treatment. It is important to note that although cancer patients may report "back pain," this pain is often complex with multifactorial etiologies, with patients needing a multidisciplinary approach to treatment.

6.1. Pain Management Strategies

To reduce back pain and minimize the impact that opioids and cancer treatment have on an individual's life, the following interventions to address back pain have potential: pharmaceutical and non-pharmacological interventions and integrative therapies. Interventions that are non-invasive and can easily be incorporated into patients' lives hold particular promise for the cancer population, and provide a more comprehensive treatment approach to pain as part of their cancer care and beyond. There are various interventions that could directly or indirectly help to mitigate back pain and are discussed below, demonstrating promise in the management of back pain in general.

In addition to reversing or stabilizing the causes of pain that may contribute to patients' back pain experience, there are several different pain management strategies to treat existing pain. In research studies, the following pain management strategies have been shown to reduce pain and improve pain-related function for individuals with cancer: pharmaceutical pain management, including medications to treat back pain and oral narcotics; non-pharmacological interventions such as physical therapy, counseling or psychotherapy, lymphedema treatment, exercise, or acupuncture; integrative therapies, including therapies and techniques that aim to affect a person's body, mind, and spirit such as meditation, yoga, tai chi, or qi gong. These techniques may have a targeted muscle or body focus where the individual may work on a specific issue, such as back pain. Pain management strategies were not consistently used by participants in the MAP. Therefore, based on pain trajectory group, the type of approach to pain management can vary between individuals and may, through subgroup analysis, be found helpful in reducing pain over time and increasing the quality of life for such patients.

6.2. Physical Therapy and Rehabilitation

Balague and colleagues studied the oncological rehabilitation system, including back and neck pain rehabilitation, and listed recommendations for the design of rehabilitation programs when treating patients with cancer-derived back pain. While exercising the patient is possible at any stage of breast cancer treatment, techniques and recommendations to consider when working with this population include minimizing activities requiring raising the hands above the head until at least 4-6 weeks after surgery, no heavy lifting on the arm involved with breast surgery, elevating the arm above the level of the shoulder to stretch the chest, once cleared, beginning stretching exercises with physical therapy and using free weights that range from 1.0 pounds to about 5.0 pounds. Strength training with free weights should begin at 4.0 pounds moving up to a maximum weight of 12.0-15.0 pounds. For breast cancer-related back pain, free weights are utilized either sitting or standing with the weights at shoulder height, keeping the elbows bent at a 90° angle while squeezing the shoulder blades together, then slowly lowering the arms, repeating 10-15 reps for one set.

Physical therapy and rehabilitation are non-invasive interventions that are utilized to manage back pain related to cancer. In physical therapy interventions, the targeted muscles for exercise and stretches include the abdominal muscles, back muscles, and hips. Yoga and Pilates also offer exercise routine options specifically targeting these muscle areas, in addition to addressing balance, coordination, directed breathing, and relaxation. Techniques in these disciplines may be used to release muscle tension and reduce the perception of back pain related to cancer. From a general exercise perspective, the three main muscle groups for back pain include the abdominal, back, and hip muscles. Additionally, for those with breast cancer, the muscle groups around the chest should also be targeted.

7. Research Studies and Case Reports

The World Health Organization estimates that there are over 20 million new cases of cancer diagnosed each year around the world. The etiology of a number of cancers includes inflammatory processes and related lifestyle factors such as obesity and physical inactivity, which are also related to nonspecific musculoskeletal pain. This chapter outlines research studies and case reports that provide an evidence base as to how the profession might understand the relationship between any upper back pain presented to a healthcare professional or manual therapist and cancer. The evidence for this chapter includes the latest research studies and reviews that offer clinical information. In addition, results from empirical studies and qualitative research have been included as this chapter develops. Overall, this chapter will examine the recent developments in understanding the signs and management of this devastating condition.

Patients with upper back pain and no obvious injury or following a traumatic event frequently seek care from primary care providers and manual therapists. An underlying more significant disease, such as cancer, can initiate pain in this region prior to becoming symptomatic elsewhere. That is why there is a very high level of interest from patients and healthcare professionals to understand the relationship between upper back pain and cancer. Cancer is a multifactorial disease where symptoms have the ability to differ greatly between patients. It is important, therefore, to search for signs and symptoms to help 'flag' that this may be a possibility requiring further investigations, such as additional imaging.

8. Conclusion and Future Directions in Research

Highlighting one unequivocal element that reveals that back pain is a product of cancer directly causing some pathological change in the vertebra is impossible due to the mixed findings of the research literature. Because of this, the recommendation for future research is that advances in neuroimaging technology will make it crucial to investigate the phenomena of the body part specific pain experiences of cancer patients. Moreover, it is recommended to investigate not only the skeletal pain experience due to cancer in the upper back, but also possible musculoskeletal pain in that area due to altered kinematics and posture. Finally, it is suggested pursuing clinical direction by examining if and which interventions are successful in reducing these diagnosed 'needless' pains and the impact on a variety of quality of life indicators.

1. Explains the methodology for performing the essay, in particular the modules used in the literature review. 2. Offers the results of the implemented search step, including the number of articles found from the databases and from other sources. 3. Provides and discusses the results of the assessment, which includes issues like study samples, cancer types, chronicity of the back pain, involved structures and the use of the most appropriate statistics. 4. Offers further insights regarding descriptive data about the reviewed research studies, including the year of publication, sample characteristics, cancer site, and main

outcome. 5. Considers major limitations like the possible publication bias in this field of research, which would render the results less conclusive.

The present article has the following features:

Exploring the Causes and Treatment of Upper Back Pain

1. Introduction to Upper Back Pain

Interest in disordered musculoskeletal pain is often stimulated by the desire to improve current knowledge and to make efforts to reach optimal therapeutic gain. Furthermore, upper back pain may significantly change an individual's neurophysiological and motor patterns. If a better understanding could be gained about musculoskeletal etiology or leg pain, it would provide information regarding those most at risk and could lead to a better understanding of the types of intervention that would be most likely to be successful. The aim of this article is to provide an overview of upper back pain, including a discussion of its etiology, presented within the context of a skilled clinical approach. The following review, aimed to establish a definition of primary back pain, has failed to identify a group of individuals purely representing the so-called "normal" back. All groups described weaknesses in muscle function significantly contributing to excessive lower back movement and pain.

While back pain is something that is episodic and temporary for most, it is experienced on a daily basis by approximately 40% of people. Research has also found that existing back pain is likely to subsequently lead to leg pain in 6-8% of cases. Long-term musculoskeletal back pain has previously been associated with the severity of depression, with scores in cases of severe depression that were far higher than those for people who had a mild level of back pain or no back pain. Upper back pain is not as common as lower back pain, but it still affects 10-12% of the population at some stage in their lives. Difficulty in the provision of treatment has left more than half of the population living with chronic musculoskeletal pain.

1.1. Anatomy of the Upper Back

With the nucleus known, the back muscles that run from the base of the head to the coccyx can be discussed. Many of the bones in the upper back are protected with muscles. The muscles then continue moving down close to the bone to the sacrum for optimal mobility and protection. In all, the muscles in the left and right connect the spine from the base of the neck and similar locations in the back, and medial portion to muscle tissues on the upper arms, shoulder blades, ribcage, and pelvis. In the top portion of the thoracic spinal column, many of these muscles are designed to rotate and pull the spinal column, which can make head, neck, and shoulder movement painful. As spine muscles extend inferiorly or synthetically that surrounds below the shoulder blade eventually covering the sacroiliac joints muscles commonly change to flexion.

In addition to the thoracic region, the upper back further contains the scapulothoracic region. This is where the scapula bone moves across the thoracic cavity. The scapula serves as a large central point for those muscles that make up the shoulder girdle complex. The muscles that stabilize and move the scapula are important for upper back function. Fused to the upper thoracic vertebrae, the upper back consists of the 12 vertebrae located behind the chest and abdomen. It is formed from thoracic vertebrae, the bones of the thorax, the thoracic cage's 12 pairs of ribs (alongside their cartilage), and the breastbone. These elements secure the spinal cord and allow you to elevate the chest and bend the thoracic spine in shoulders, which is quite a limited range of motion (ROM) and allows for nothing but 15-20° of thoracic extension and just a small amount of flexion. With the help of strengthening exercises that target these posterior chain muscles, the movement of the thoracic spine can be maintained and the upper back can be strengthened.

The upper back comprises the thoracic area consisting of 12 vertebrae. This portion of the spine is tasked with the ribcage's primary function of protecting many important organs such as the heart, the lungs, the liver, as well as the spleen. The cervical region may be the most mobile portion of the spine, with many muscles assisting in the numerous movements it can execute. The upper back, like the thoracic area in the torso, comprises twelve vertebrae. This part of the spine is in charge of protecting the ribcage and the thoracic cavity's essential organs. These bones grow more extensive as they move inferiorly. Each time the bone arises, it connects to a pair of stabilizing ribs to complete an anatomical circle known through facets. Throughout this sequence, the facets progress, turning the spine circular orientation these bones grow wider/distally. Consequently, this placement warrants a stiffer design for the lower and middle back segment which is typified by the ribcage support system.

The upper back is a complex part of the body. It is made up of the thoracic spine, which is comprised of 12 vertebrae. The thoracic spine is connected to the cervical spine at the base and the lumbar spine at the bottom. Once we travel to the front of the torso, the thoracic spine includes a series of 12 rib pairs on each side that assist in forming the chest area, keeping important organs safe. The shoulder girdle is also a part of the upper back, running from the arm to thoracic, and containing bones, including the scapula and clavicle, as well as ligaments and cartilage. Extending from the cervical vertebrae, which lie deep within the neck, to the base of the ribcage, which forms the thoracic spine, these bones run from the cervical vertebrae in the neck to the base of the 12 rib pairs of the thoracic cavity in the torso. Each vertebra is attached to the others by muscles, articulating facet joints, and tendons. The sternum makes up the anterior aspect of the spine in the upper trunk, forming the initial costovertebral and costosternal joints. The thoracic portion, including the upper back, is not designed for flexibility but primarily for anchoring the ribcage and its movements.

2. Common Causes of Upper Back Pain

Posture and Muscle Strain. Posture is another common, overlooked cause of upper back pain. As technology has advanced and people can work, game, and communicate with one another right from where they are, they are more often dependent on the use of electrical or electronic devices for extended periods of time. This includes leaning and bending the head and neck forward, such as when using a smartphone, computer workstation, gaming system, or repeatedly looking down while watching television. As opposed to standing up straight with the ears aligned with the shoulders, which is suggested by the Centre for Disease Control and Prevention (CDC), this posture can cause or exacerbate pain in the upper back. In a similar vein to patient-reported outcomes, existing clinical practice guidelines help physicians determine what interventions are suitable for patients based on the results of studies conducted on various groups.

Upper back pain is a common condition that impacts individuals of all backgrounds and ages. Nonetheless, experts have established several typical causes of upper back pain. The leading triggers of upper back pain typically influence lifestyle, including the sort of tasks in which one partakes, stature, and exposure to disorder and/or traumatic life events. The most common triggers of upper back pain include muscle strain or sprain and poor posture. However, other key causes include the wear and tear of spinal discs over time, disc herniations that compress nearby nerves, and pinched or compressed nerves. Other ailments that affect the spine or its surrounding tissues, such as scoliosis, infection, arthritis, and fractures, also often induce pain in the upper back.

2.1. Muscle Strain and Sprain

Muscle strain is perhaps the most common source of back pain, either between the shoulder blades or up the entire back. The fibers in muscles tear in response to unaccustomed activity: for example, unscrewing a cap or raking leaves after winter hibernation, which has made the muscles too forceful in an effort to overcome stiffness or scar tissue from previous injuries. This may be intensified by poor posture and muscle tone, localized muscle spasms, calcifications, or bone spurs that have become irritants, and wider problems that change the way these muscles operate. The difference between a strain and a sprain is rather subtle: it comes down to whether tendons and/or muscles are affected. Tendons are fibrous bands that connect the muscles to the bones; ligaments are also fibrous bands, but they connect bone to bone. The expected time for recovery and recurrence rates are largely determined by the length of tenderness and strength deficits: if the tenderness lasts 10 days, there is usually a significant muscle injury; if pain and strength deficits last six weeks, there is usually organic damage to either muscle or bone, or to the mechanism of nervous control of strength.

There are a number of causes of upper back problems, but muscle strain and sprain are the most common. When movement occurs, we ask our muscles to engage, but if we sustain a force that exceeds what the muscles can withstand, muscles and tendons become damaged: tears, strains, and even ruptures are possible. Most commonly, the upper back becomes injured when one level of the spine becomes too rigid to absorb the forces of movement. The thoracic spine itself is typically immobile, protected by the ribcage, which makes it unlikely to suffer the same microscopic damage of repetitive movements that the cervical and lumbar spine so often do. Instead, upper back pain often occurs as a result of problems in the cervical and/or lumbar spine which place stress on the muscles of the thoracic spine. The upper back protects the nerves of the spinal cord as they travel from the brain to the peripheries of the body. Arthritis, inflammation, disc displacement, fractures, and other structural problems may cause compression of the nerves or nerves to protective muscles, leading to spasm and upper back pain.

2.2. Poor Posture

A slouched posture impacts the natural S-shaped curve of the spine. It also forces the head forward, which puts extra pressure on the neck. Long-term poor posture can cause upper back pain, especially when a person is in one position for long periods of time. If bad habits, such as poor seated posture, are not rectified, then the pain will not go away because the area becomes inflamed. Posture exercises and stretches are important for upper back pain treatment and prevention. By doing these along with the right posture, you will be able to minimize discomfort.

Persons who set themselves up for poor posture are those who use the computer for long periods of time. These people are often in pain because typically they will be leaning forward and not against the back of the chair. This causes the shoulders to hunch forward and down, with the head leaning down, not fully supported by the headrests. Because the muscles in the upper back and neck are infrequently used for long periods, the muscles fatigue. A flatter headrest on a chair will also limit neck support and force a scrunched position on the neck, upper back, and shoulder muscles, which can be very uncomfortable. A good quality upper back support is very important if a person is going to avoid muscle strain and pain. Good posture also means going through the correct motions with minimal strain and energy exertion.

The most common culprit of upper back pain is poor posture. Every joint from the top of our neck to the bottom of our body should have an ideal biomechanical position. When we slouch with our upper backs hunched forward, the muscles that are naturally taut and serve as a back brace become over-stretched and weakened. The body's reaction is to deposit sticky, fibrous tissue in the weakened areas, such as the upper portion of the back, resulting in small restrictions and stiffness to develop in the muscles and fascia. Prolonged imbalance of postural muscles is not only associated with pain mechanisms but secures a perpetuating cycle of discomfort.

3. Less Common Causes of Upper Back Pain

Degenerative disc disease technically affects the whole spine, but it more commonly affects the lumbar spine – probably because there are five discs in the lumbar spine and fewer in the thoracic spine. Although degenerative disc disease usually leads to pain at the specific level of the spine, which is the lumbar or lower back most of the time, this phenomenon shows that other causes of thoracic pain include spondylolisthesis – a spinal disorder that involves forward slippage of one or more of the lower lumbar vertebrae relative to the upper vertebrae. Juvenile, or adolescent, spondylolisthesis develops between the ages of 12 and 15, and adult spondylolisthesis tends to become a problem around age 40. It is 10 times less likely to afflict adult women than adult men and, interestingly, it is not any easier to treat, surgically or otherwise, than juvenile spondylolisthesis.

Expert's advice: "Rare" causes of upper back pain. Less common, but still relevant, sources of upper back pain tend to afflict people in specific age ranges, and in some cases, there is an overlap between causes also being risk factors. Some of the causes of upper, but not lower, thoracic or lumbosacral back pain include degenerative disc disease that affects various levels of the spine. Nurse Email Address: carolinep@gundersenhealth.org, licensed practical nurse and PhD candidate (Applied Clinical

Informatics) at the University of Wisconsin-Madison School of Nursing.

3.1. Degenerative Disc Disease

A person with degenerative disc disease may experience a grating sensation, joint swelling, or acute ongoing pain that's intense enough to wake them up at night. There are also problems with muscle strain as the body tries to compensate for the ongoing discomfort. The upper back may even round or the entire spine can appear twisted. The progression of degenerative disc disease varies; treatment isn't aimed at halting the progress of the illness, as there are no real advancements in stopping the sort of damage that occurs with DDD. Instead, doctors work to minimize back pain.

Symptoms of Degenerative Disc Disease

Degenerative disc disease is another potential reason those with upper back pain seek medical care. Degenerative disc disease itself occurs when the discs in the upper back seem to age irregularly. Though a part of the aging process, not everyone experiences pain as a result of the changes in their discs. One of the most common causes of upper back pain, degenerative disc disease changes the discs of the upper back. Located between the vertebral bones, the discs serve to act as cushions or shock absorbers for the bones that make up the spine. When injuries or accidents occur in this area, these spongy discs can become damaged. Unlike cartilage in other parts of the body, the discs of the upper back contain very few blood vessels, which can complicate the healing process.

4. When to Seek Medical Attention

- Symptoms including chest pain, nausea, fatigue, appetite reduction, osteoporosis, a family background of severe diseases, leg weakness, tremor, extraordinary body or limb strength, and disturbance on one hand of the man's genitalia, specifically the scrotum. Consequently, she vehemently debilitated my calf pain and unreasonably debilitated my hind. Foot drop, or paresthesias or digestive discomfort (for instance, the inability to remove your nerves), may affect you having to treat other illnesses including spinal adjustment, osteopenia, poor friend activity, pre-existing intervertebral disc disease (including metastasis or eocles glue) and many eastern countries that can slow the blood flow. Even for physician or hospital visits, allowance or hearing/management. These are called "dislocations," and they can affect the type and degree of treatment that is encouraged. If you suddenly develop persistent diarrhea, malnutrition causes mass losses, which are sometimes severe, through the anal hypertension [or are] called "cauda equina syndrome and "unseen" instantiation, which typically has extreme lower extremities and also has bowel or ampoule problems, and also has or does have religious impact, this is a method of decision that requires our attention. In the third set, post-frequency proportion compression occurs, as well as rods or a process (cluster) disorder, in which well-being can lead to a cardiovascular incident. Classic features can involve the onset of pain between now and then a few years, in tandem with a gradual increase in the body and the point at which analgesics are ineffective. Conversely, steel reinforced knee osteoarthritis.

The following are regarded as red flags:

A recent injury or a natural progression of degenerative conditions can lead to discomfort in the upper back. The condition is generally not serious, requiring a few days of rest or at-home treatments. However, knowing when to visit a doctor for back pain is critical. Understanding the signs of serious health problems and the signs of a true emergency can save your health.

4.1. Red Flags for Serious Conditions

• >8/10 pain in 20-30 minute intervals without relief • Numbness, pins and needles, or weakness in upper extremities • A >8/10 pain during coughing, sneezing, or bowel movement • Constant dull or aching pain • Pain often happens at night and is worse when lying down or resting • Pain not improving with 2 to 4 weeks of conservative treatment such as medications and physical therapy • Pain increases when body temperature increases (fever, chills) because of an infection • Pain resulting from an existing or recent serious impact could cause fractures, dislocations, ligamentous injuries, and structural or neurological deficits

The sites at which upper back pain occurs the most include the shoulder blades, spine, rib cage, and base of the neck. Because of this, pain in this area usually stems from problems with those aforementioned structures. It is also possible that pain referred from the stomach, gallbladder, or heart may be felt in this area. In more severe cases, you should immediately seek medical attention for your condition. Some signs of a potentially higher-risk issue being behind the pain include:

5. Diagnosis of Upper Back Pain

Electrical testing of the speed of the nerves can also be used by a professional. When analyzed collectively, physical testing findings can assist your healthcare provider in diagnosing your discomfort. This is referred to as the "diagnosis." Blood testing is rarely performed to confirm or exclude the source of your back pain. It can be used, for example, to confirm a diagnosis of a rheumatological disorder such as ankylosing spondylitis or an immune-related condition like lupus. A precise diagnosis is the first step in effective back pain care. It is through this process that a doctor can discover the source of your discomfort. It will be capable of successfully treating your discomfort, avoiding future occurrences, and outlining the best treatment.

Multiple types of healthcare providers offer diagnostic services for back pain, including general practitioners, chiropractors, and orthopedic specialists. During a physical examination, your doctor or therapist will obtain your medical history and discuss your symptoms with you. They will palpate or feel your muscle tissue, ligaments, and vertebrae to ascertain the cause of discomfort. This also enables them to detect regions of inflammation or muscle spasms and evaluate your range of motion. If additional diagnosis is needed, your doctor can use x-rays, magnetic resonance imaging (MRI), or computed tomography (CT) scans.

5.1. Physical Examination

If trigger points are suspected, the location of tenderness may be elicited by touching parts of the musculature, rather than the bones. In maximal tenderness lacking discernible locations, digital pressure is applied in a rotary manner over muscle bellies at the previously mentioned anatomical landmarks. Postural evaluation is achieved by having the patient stand comfortably in a normal sagittal orientation. The examiner then observes the plumb line position. This is a psychological reference line that is directed through the external auditory canal, the acromion processes, and the sacrum. Each of these three structures should be bilaterally symmetrical. After checking these relationships, the examiner notes where the "center of gravity" is in relation to the feet. If the sagittal line in front of the external auditory canal is immediately anterior to the ankle joint, then the weight is too far anterior. If it is behind the ankle, the weight is too far back. In both instances, this could be an indication of spasticity or rigidity of some of the anterior or posterior muscle chains, respectively.

A thorough physical examination can provide valuable diagnostic information regarding the cause and extent of upper back pain. It may also determine if consultation with specialists is necessary. A comprehensive examination includes postural assessment, measurement of range of motion (both active and passive), and elicitation of pain upon palpation of the intrinsic and extrinsic structures of the upper back. When performing a physical examination, the physician should be attentive to all possible sources of upper back pain including the cervical paraspinal muscles, the thoracic paraspinal muscles, the thoracic interspinous spaces, the facet joints, the costo-transverse joints, the costovertebral joints, the angle of Louis (sternomanubrial joint), the sterno-clavicular joints, the upper lumbar facet joints, the pedicles, the transverse processes, and the spinous processes from T1 to T12 level. Tenderness is tested over each of these areas, usually with the use of the physician's thumb.

5.2. Imaging Tests

- X-rays. This is usually the first test done for an unexplained upper back complaint as most causes of upper back pain are picked up with an X-ray. Often healthcare professionals will also request that you have your neck X-rayed and that the images include Flexion/Extension – forward and backward bending of the neck. - MRI (Magnetic Resonance Imaging) scans. MRI is able to provide clear pictures of the tissues surrounding the breast, in order to help healthcare professionals see the structure within the back and any abnormalities present. An MRI can pick up the same conditions as those that would show up on an X-ray and other abnormalities such as disc bulges, chronically inflamed (swollen) nerves or a stenosis (narrowing) along the spine, which can cause upper back pain. This test uses a strong magnet to produce images of the body part being examined. - Myelogram/CT scans. This special type of X-ray gives a detailed view of the bones & soft tissue in your back. During this test, a special dye is injected into your spinal canal via a lumbar puncture (injection in your lower back). As the dye moves upwards into the spine, it lights up the nerve & spinal canal. Then a CT scan is done to provide detailed images of the inside of your body. After some upper back conditions have been diagnosed, the healthcare professional will discuss with you the most appropriate form of treatment.

Several different diagnostic imaging tests might be used to assess upper back pain. The most commonly used tests to view the upper back include:

6. Treatment Options

Another treatment option is massage, which can relax the muscles in your back, and a therapist may also use heat and/or ice packs to provide relief. Heat therapy using warm towels, hot packs or a warm bath can help loosen your muscles and ease your upper back pain. Cold therapy using ice packs or a cold gel pack will help numb your upper back area, reducing pain and swelling. There are many medications that can help reduce upper back pain, including OTC pain relievers such as acetaminophen, and for more severe pain, you may be prescribed prescription-strength medications. If you have repeated episodes of upper back pain, you should practice self-care to help prevent or ease symptoms. You should also take care to practice good posture, and sit, stand, and lie in positions that don't worsen your pain. Anti-anxiety medications such as benzodiazepines can help deal with the emotional side of pain, such as anxiety or depression. You should never take any medication without consulting a healthcare provider first, as some medications can interact with each other. Orthotics can be great for prevention as well. You may want to wear shoes with well-cushioned soles or try shoe inserts as comfort padding in your shoes. These will help stop a future upper back pain episode by reducing the chances of your ribs experiencing undue pressure.

Physical therapy is a common treatment for upper back pain. You may need to start with a gentle exercise program that gets progressively more challenging as your body gets stronger and heals. A physical therapist can check your technique to make sure the exercises are safe and effective for you. Spinal manipulation is also an effective treatment for upper back pain. Your physical therapist uses their hands to apply pressure to small areas of your muscles or along your spine. The manipulation helps loosen the tight muscles in your upper back and relieve pain.

6.1. Physical Therapy

For people focusing on physical therapy from home, there are various exercises that a person can perform to build strength in the area. It can also be beneficial to try yoga, Pilates, swimming exercises, and other techniques that are designed to support the natural movement of the neck, upper back, and arms. Engaging in these sorts of exercises with good body awareness might help to prevent the onset of upper back pain by improving strength and flexibility and making a person more resistant to injury. By improving a person's posture, resistance to injury, and the overall functioning of their core, they might alleviate upper back and shoulder blade pain in the long run.

Physical therapy is a treatment that includes a range of rehabilitative techniques that can help to alleviate upper back pain, shoulder blade discomfort, and related symptoms. Physical therapy can also help to prevent the onset of pain. Physical therapy can involve using various exercises and stretches to strengthen the neck, shoulder, and upper back area. These exercises may additionally engage the use of resistance bands, weights, or resistance machines in a controlled environment. The goal of physical therapy for upper back pain is to focus on the area of symptoms from a functional perspective. Based on the individual's experience and physical findings, a physical therapist will prioritize exercises and treatment approaches. For example, focusing on exercises that strengthen postural muscles, reduce muscle tension, or improve thoracic spine mobility. The program will also include an education component, addressing items such as proper posture and how to adjust ergonomics to diminish stress on the neck and upper back. Physical therapy can also incorporate hands-on "manual" massage, soft tissue work, or utilizing modalities like electrical stimulation, dry needling, or heat to alleviate pain and soreness.

6.2. Medications

In order to reduce pain levels, your doctor may suggest over-the-counter pain relievers. Medications such as acetaminophen (Tylenol) are used to provide relief when pain is at a low or moderate level. If muscle spasms are contributing to your pain, a muscle relaxant may help. This medication works to calm muscle spasms and reduce tension. It is typically prescribed for short-term use. It may make you feel sleepy or tired, so don't take it if you have to be active and on alert. In the case of acute upper back pain, you may be prescribed a stronger medication that can be taken for relief. Anti-inflammatory drugs known as NSAIDs are prescribed to reduce inflammation, which is one of the reasons for the development of pain. Your healthcare professional will go over the advantages and disadvantages of using NSAIDs and decide which one can help you the most. ACOEM recommends that NSAIDs be approved for use in acute pain management. If you are a woman aged 50 or older or a man aged 40 or older, your healthcare professional may not want to use NSAIDs as a first-line therapy unless the benefits outweigh the risks. In some cases, the use of NSAIDs can lead to side effects in the gastrointestinal tract. Some NSAIDs can also result in an increased risk of heart attack or stroke. Your healthcare professional may suggest that you use a medication that is easier on the stomach.

Medications can help provide relief from upper back pain. Most often, healthcare professionals will recommend using medication in conjunction with non-medicinal treatment modalities to achieve the best results. As well, when mental health struggles are occurring simultaneously, medications that treat anxiety and depression may be integrated into the treatment plan prescribed by a psychiatrist.

7. Preventive Measures

Upper back pain shown on plain radiographs can be caused by several different conditions or issues. Normal aging results in degeneration of bones and discs, and radiographic images can demonstrate various mild abnormalities, including osteophytes and disc space narrowing, to severe joint space changes on images. Correlation of bone changes can relate to physical exam, history, evaluation of pain characteristics, and a focused treatment management plan. Treatment of upper back pain involves not only reducing or eliminating symptoms but also restoring function to prevent long-lasting issues. Generally, patients are offered conservative treatment options before proceeding to more invasive treatments. Exercises to stretch and improve strength and endurance, as well as developing core strength, have been found to have positive long-term benefits. Posture and muscle imbalance training have been found to be beneficial as well. Chiropractic or manipulation has been found to be beneficial as well in some cases. Injections can be done diagnostically to confirm the source of the patient's pain. Neural injections are used to determine the holy language of the upper back.

Preventive measures. Upper back problems can be prevented by avoiding risk factors. In the case of work-related problems, employers can put ergonomic workstations and related education into place. This study strongly suggests that an appropriate workstation is important for preventing upper back pain. First, the height of the workstation should not be so high that the user lifts their shoulders or tenses the upper trapezius muscles when working. Second, the height of the computer display and the keyboard should be set so that workers do not look downward or upward while working. Third, workers using digital devices should take regular breaks because they are both static and dynamic. Musculoskeletal problems are multifactorial conditions, incorporating physical, psychological, and social components. Additionally, they are often recurrent. Interactions between different risk factors over time ultimately cause the prevalence of initial episodes and recurrence. Good postural habits and a proper workstation could also play a role in minimizing the likelihood of developing upper back pain.

7.1. Ergonomic Workstations

It is most important for everyone to sit in a high-back chair, with the low back resting against the lower lumbar support, to provide a good base of support. The natural S-shaped posture of the lower back should be maintained while sitting with the legs at a 90-degree angle. If the chair does not have proper lower back support, it is possible to use a pillow placed between the chair back and the person's mid-back. At the same time, proper keyboard usage actually encourages good upper back posture and shoulder stability. The first important point in positioning the keyboard is to shift the sheath of the wrist slightly forward. Sit back in an office chair far enough as recommended and then bend the elbow at a 90-degree angle. The hands should normally sit with a straight forearm and a straight line, referring to when the person pushes the hand forward, while the knees rest just below the elbows. Second, the computer monitor's position should be aligned with the person's eye level. This means that the computer screen should be at eye level. The computer screen is sometimes positioned too high or too low, causing the head and neck to move unnaturally. Ergonomic desks and workstations should be arranged in the most useful and efficient way to alleviate pain. Additionally, it is essential to customize the keyboard mechanisms to suit the individual's needs. Ergonomic office workstations offer unique settings for each user. Ensure that the work materials are organized properly to facilitate productivity and reduce strain. Take breaks every hour to relax and stretch. Performing gravity swings or aerobic exercises can help relax the shoulders and feet. It is beneficial to stand or move around at least once every hour while sitting to counteract the negative effects of prolonged sitting. Exercise is therefore crucial in preventing conditions like spondylolisthesis. Prolonged sitting can overload the muscles and cause them to stop firing properly. Muscles need sufficient energy to function properly, so it is important to avoid prolonged sitting.

Ergonomic workstations

Two of the major causes of upper back pain that can be controlled are the chair and keyboard used for work or leisure.

7. Ergonomic Equipment - Chair and Keyboard

7.1 Ergonomic Workstations

8. Conclusion and Future Directions

An effective approach to addressing the epidemic of upper back pain in colonized people, which leads to illness, work loss, and sometimes premature death, is the decolonization of white settler-colonial culture and society. A future exploratory venture may involve querying a broad cross-section of the affected population to record the ways in which white settler-colonial culture and society lead to upper back pain. This could result in the identification of physical and psychological causes beyond those discovered during this literature review. Further research may look into how white settler-colonialism affects the intervention and treatment undertaken for upper back pain to assess where there is potential for doing better.

This essay sought to provide an overview of the causes of and potential treatments for upper back pain in colonized and historically marginalized people. Upper back pain in this population stems from structural factors such as imbalance in corporeal asymmetry, poor posture, and the dominant physicality and stress from living in a white settler-colonial nation. Upper back pain can also arise from non-structural causes such as psychological stress and anxiety. It can be treated using physical therapies such as massage, chiropractic, and physical therapy, as well as biomedical treatments including anatomy and pain physiology education advertisements, drugs such as nonsteroidal anti-inflammatory drugs, muscle relaxers, and opioids, and surgeries such as discectomy and foraminotomy.

www.ingramcontent.com/pod-product-compliance
Lightning Source LLC
Chambersburg PA
CBHW071103260726

48661CB00006B/2427